Homemade Lip Balm:

30 Natural Lip Balm Recipes To Nourish, Rejuvenate And Protect Your Lips

Table of content:

Introduction

Lip balm is what they call in another term, lip salve. It is the substance you want to apply on your lips when they feel dry and chapped. Often too, lip balm is used when someone has angular cheilitis or stomatitis; or is just suffering from cold sores. Incidentally, what is this cheilitis? Well, it is another term given to chapping of lips, only this time the chapping is significantly severe. In fact, you get to see real cracks around your lip corners. Sometimes, however, cheilitis is caused by infection, and so if your lip balm does not seem to work, you better ask your doctor what the heck is happening to your lips. In short, we are saying here that lip balm, lovely as it is for your comfort and beauty, is not a substitute for medication.

There are certain seasons of the year that dry out your lips. Think winter for sure, and even changes between seasons like winter to spring, summer to fall, and fall to winter. No one likes chapped lips. They are tender, dry and can be sensitive.

Walk down the cosmetic aisle in any store, and you will see a grand display of lip balms, chap sticks, and other lip potions. Have you considered what ingredients are used? These balms go on your lips. Consider if the ingredients are chemicals, petroleum-based and may do more harm than good. Do you want to have artificial flavors and colors on your lips?

Since this is your mouth, we know that some of what you put on your lips will be ingested. It makes great sense to make your lip balms.

Chapter 1 – Main Ingredients Used in making the Homemade Lip Balms.

Here is the list of the many ingredients you will need for these recipes.

You can buy these essential oils at your local health food store. Or you can purchase them directly from essential oil companies.

Honey

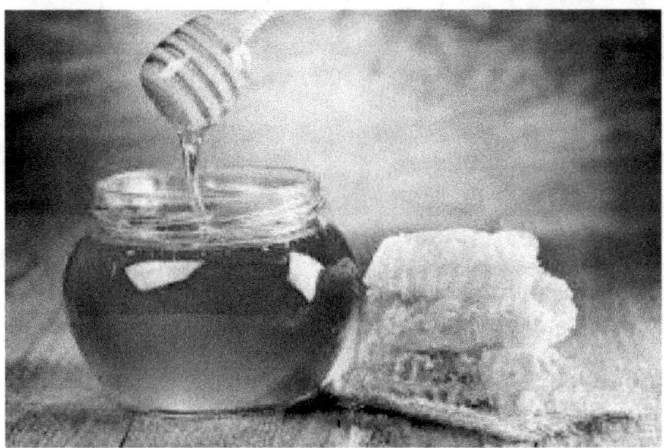

Honey is an excellent natural ingredient that contains healing and antibacterial properties that can heal damaged skin, including chapped lips.

1.   Simply, apply a teaspoon of pure organic honey onto your chapped lips two times a day.

2.   Apply before going to bed to enjoy soft lips when you wake up.

Rose Petals

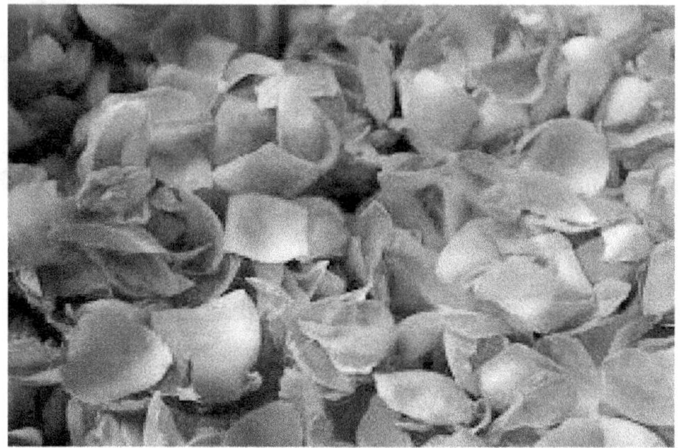

A rose plant can come to rescue when one must endure chapped lips. Rose petals can maintain your lip's moisture and can also enhance its beautiful natural color.

1.   Wash a handful of rose petals in lukewarm water.

2.   Allow the rose petals to soak in almond milk or coconut milk for two hours or more. This is to enhance the rose petals properties.

3.   With a masher or a fork, mash the rose petals into a thick paste.

4.   Apply the rose petal paste on your chapped lips two to three times a day and every night before you go to sleep.

Coconut Oil

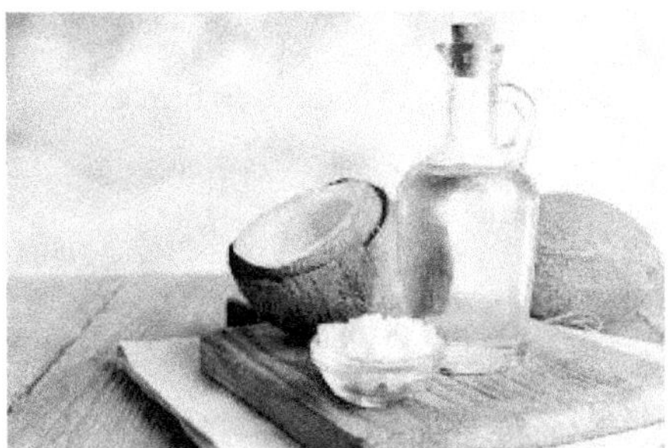

Another fabulous ingredient that can help renew and heal chapped lips is through the inherent powers that carry in coconut oil. All that you need to do is apply a teaspoon of pure coconut oil onto your lips three times a day.

Castor Oil

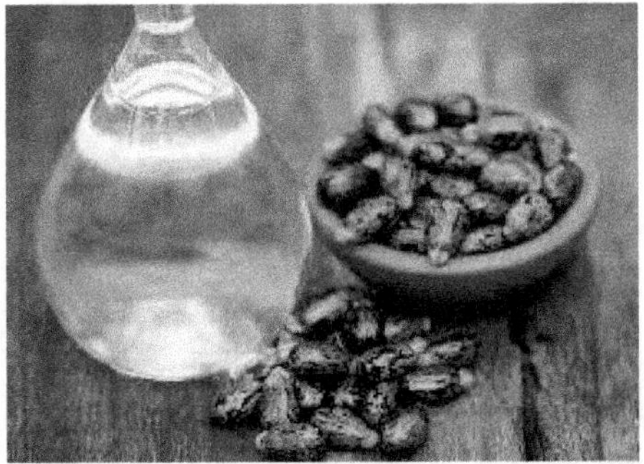

Castor oil is another natural oil that can help heal dry and chapped lips. In the same manner with the coconut oil treatment, apply castor oil to your lips one to three times a day. Alternatively, you can create a castor oil paste onto your lips.

1.   In a bowl, mix a teaspoon of castor oil, a teaspoon of glycerin, and a few drops of fresh lemon juice.

2.   Mix it well and apply it on your lips before going to bed. Do not rinse.

3.   In the morning, wash it off with a wet cotton ball.

4.   Simply apply castor oil to your lips several times a day.

5.   Repeat this treatment daily until your lips are healed.

Milk Cream

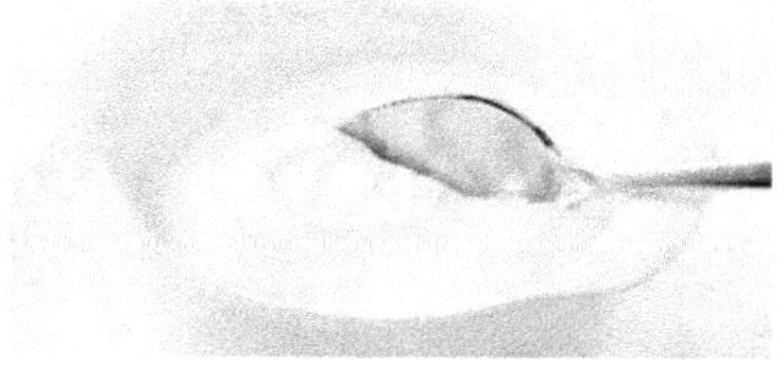

Milk cream has antibacterial and inflammatory properties making it an outstanding moisturizer for treating your lips.

1.   All that you need to do is apply fresh milk cream onto your lips.

2.   Leave it on for ten to twenty minutes.

3.   Wash your lips gently with a cotton ball.

4.   Repeat daily for the best of results.

Aloe Vera Gel

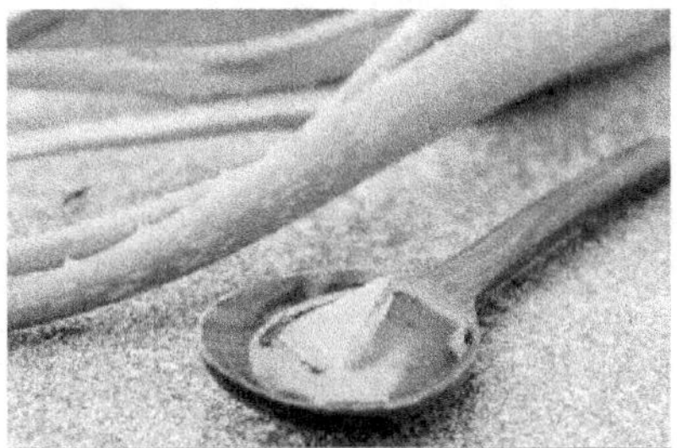

Aloe Vera gel has intense healing properties. Just by applying a small amount of Aloe Vera gel on your lips daily, it can help heal and relieve the pain from chapped lips.

Cucumber

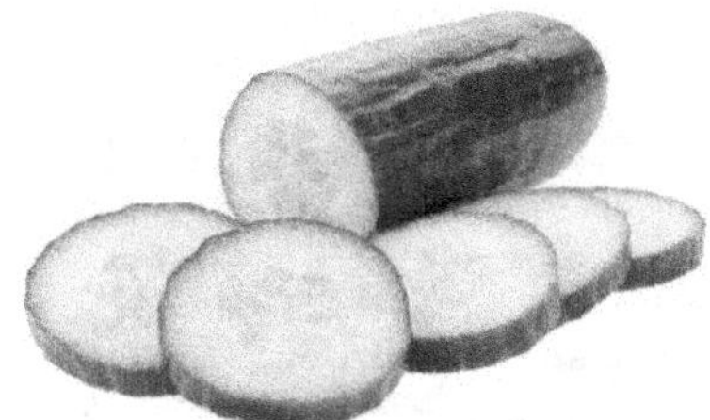

Another true answer on how to treat your chapped lips are through the natural powers of cucumbers. Here is how you can do this:

1.   Cut a fresh organic cucumber into small slices.

2.   Rub a thinly slice piece of cucumber across your chapped lips. Make sure that the juice is applied to the mouth.

3.   Leave the cucumber juice in your mouth for 15 to 20 minutes.

4.   Wash your lips with lukewarm water and apply moisturizer.

5.   Repeat daily to help your lips heal faster.

Petroleum Jelly

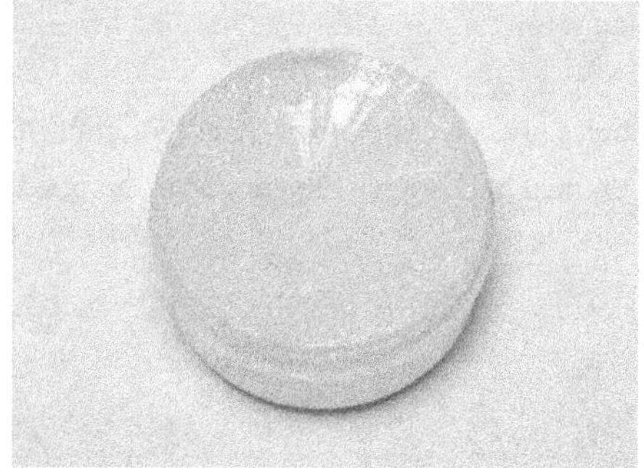

Petroleum jelly is very effective in treating your dry and chapped lips. All you need to do is apply some pure petroleum jelly over your chapped lips several times throughout your day to keep them well protected and moisturized. Before you go to sleep reapply more petroleum jelly to keep your lips moisturized and nourished overnight.

Water

Dehydration is a primary reason behind chapped and dry lips. Thus, it is imperative to drink plenty of water throughout the day to keep your body well hydrated. Try drinking about eight glasses of water every day. Not only water can keep you well-hydrated, but water can flush toxins out of your body and bring greater health overall.

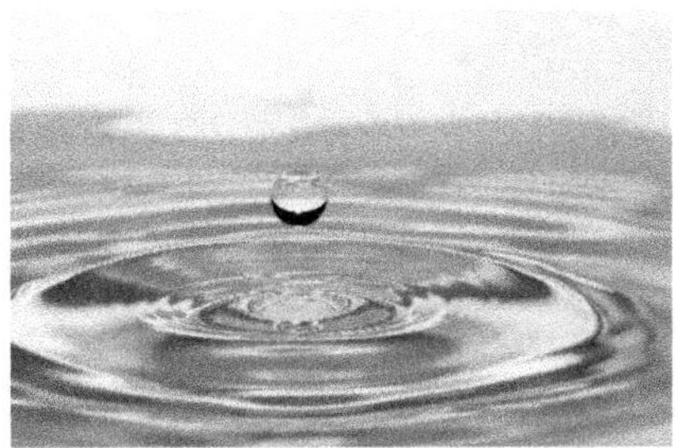

Now, these remedies are only useful if you want to treat your dry and chapped lips. These natural ingredients can also prevent them from coming back and keep them well-nourished. If you use these ingredients daily, avoid harsh weathers, eat healthily, and keep your lips well moisturized, then for sure dry lips will be gone.

Beeswax

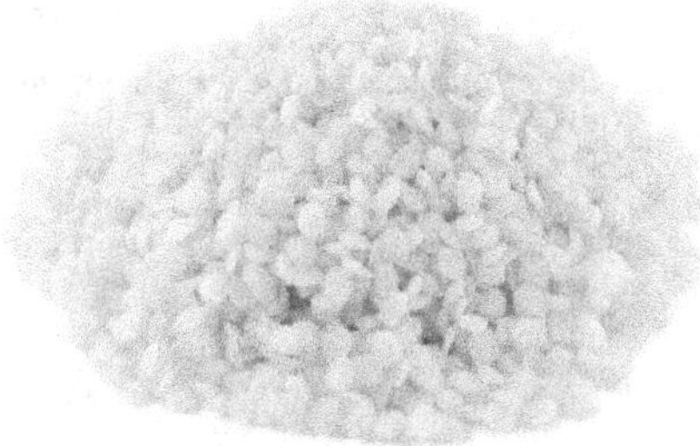

Beeswax is a natural compound product used in many cosmetics today. It can be very moisturizing and be used to help protect your lips from the harmful rays of the sun. It also contains natural emulsifiers, which can help retain the moisture in your skin. This makes beeswax an essential ingredient in most lip balm.

Carrier Oils

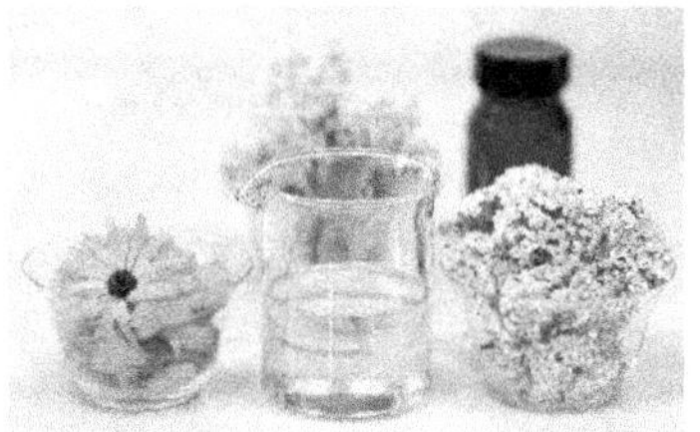

Also, called base oils. Carrier oils are simply vegetable oils; they are used to dilute the concentrate essential oils before applied to the skin. Therefore, carrier oils are useful to mix with essential oils because it is sometimes necessary to dilute them to the appropriate concentration to use on the skin. Carrier oils help in absorption and not too easy to evaporate.

These are some of the carrier oils used in lip balm you can choose by your preference; they don't make much different in the result products except a slightly different smell.

Rosehip Seed Oil

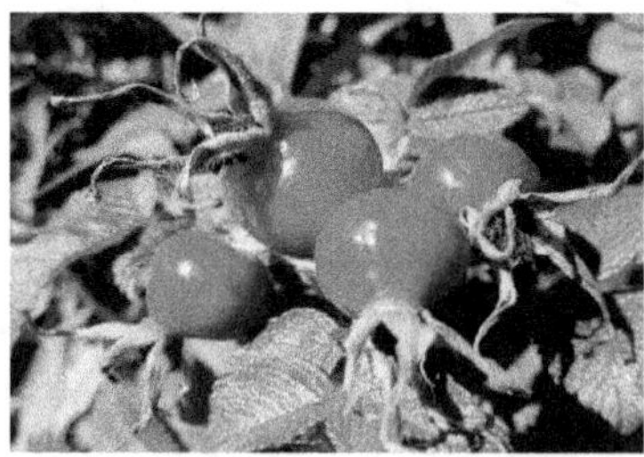

Rosehip seed oil is an excellent moisturizer and has wonderful properties for the skin, especially to cure conditions due to scarring and sun damage.

Calendula Oil

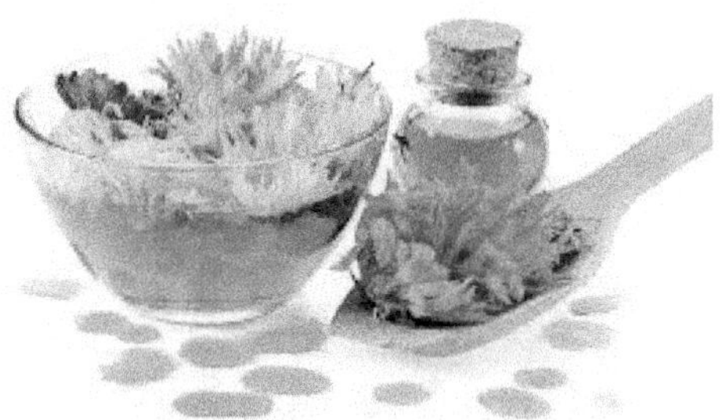

Calendula oil has anti-inflammatory properties that can soften and soothe your lips, thus making it useful in healing several skin conditions. It also can treat irritated skin, remove dead skins, and promote new skin cell growth.

Wheat Germ Oil

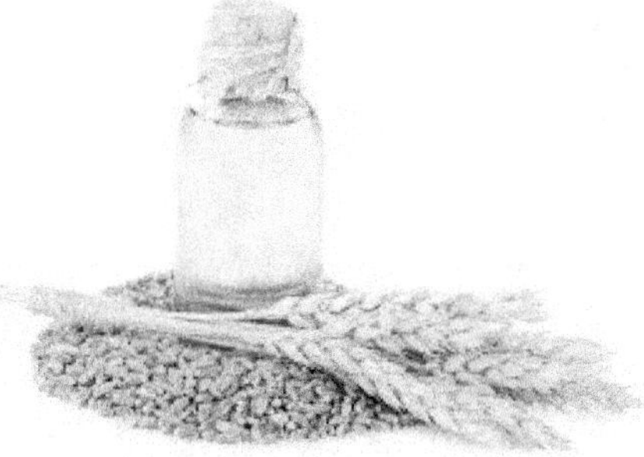

Wheat germ oil has natural antioxidants such as Vitamin and Beta Carton; it is popular to be used in skin care product because of its mild odor and specific ability to easily spread on the skin.

Avocado Oil

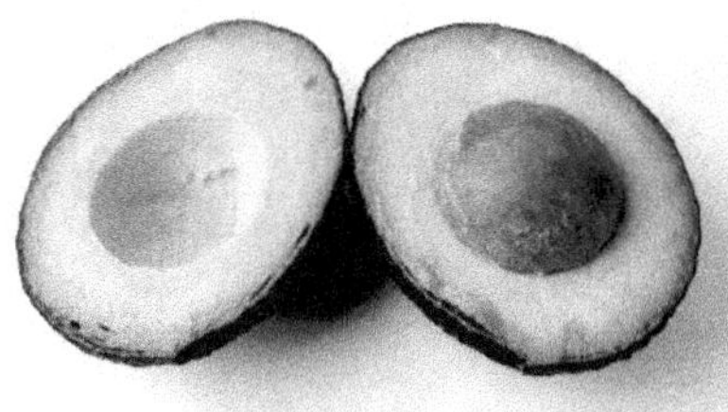

Avocado Oil is rich in proteins, fatty acids, and many vitamins, including A, D, E, B1, B2, and B5. Avocado oil also contains properties that can provide ultraviolet protection to shield your lips from the harmful rays of the sun. Avocado oil also leaves you with softening and smooth lips after use.

Almond Oil

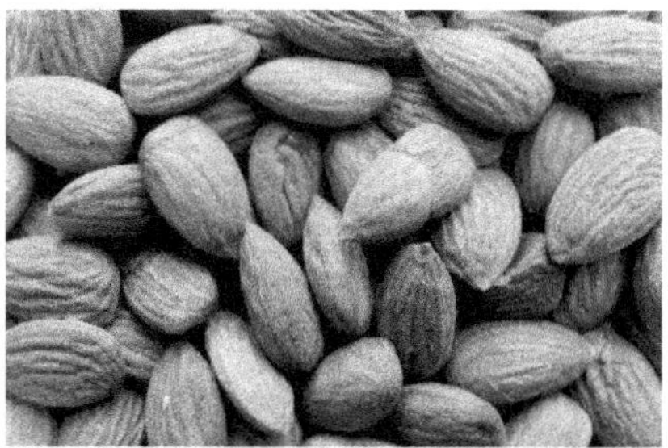

Almond oil is one of the most favorites of carrier oils. This oil contains softening abilities coming from essential fatty acids and vitamins A, E, B1, B2, and B6. Almond oil also has a softening capacity and can help protect and nourish your lips.

Olive Oil

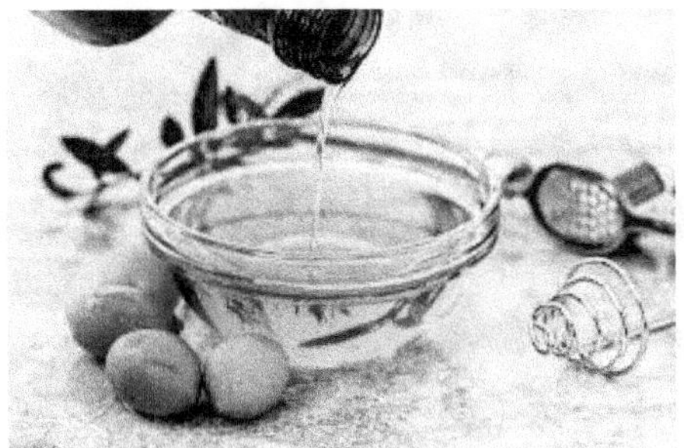

Olive oil is rich in Vitamin E, a soothing skin moisturizer with healing properties. Used as a conditioner and a moisturizer and very compatible with all skin types.

Sunflower Oils

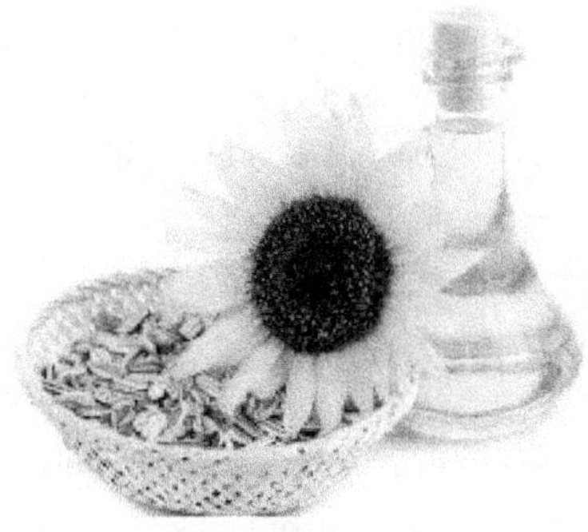

Sunflower oil is an essential fatty acid in which it is high in vitamin E. Sunflower oil also works for all skin types; it can treat dry skin, aging skin, and damaging skin.

Essential Oils

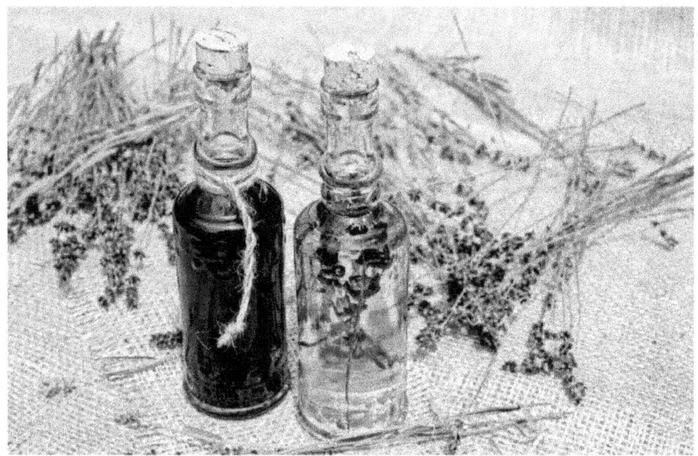

Essential oils are distilled from aromatic plants including the leave, flower, bark, and roots. These essential oils to the lip balms to create the pleasant odors and tactile sensations. For example, rose essential oil has a floral scent like the lip applied with a real rose all the time, grapefruit essential oil has fruit, citrus-like odor, gives the refreshing feeling, and the addition of peppermint essential oil can cause a pleasantly tingling sensation on the lips.

Different essential oils provide different effects on our mood, for example, rose essential oil gives relaxing feelings, grapefruit, essential oil makes the mood refreshing, and perming essential oil has stimulating action.

Natural color

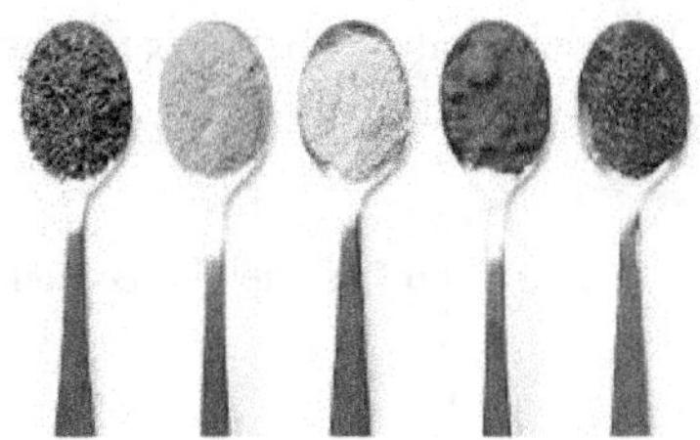

Natural colors are natural dyeing agents made from ground up plants parts or herbs such as petals, leaves, root, bark, pollen, *etc.* and has a wide range of different shades, depending on how concentrated. These are some popular natural powder color you can use as lip color pigment or tint.

Beetroot powder – light pink color to deep purple color
Ground turmeric – yellow
Sandalwood red powder – red
Spinach powder – green
Raspberry powder – light red to deep red, light pink
Ground rose petals – light pink, red
Alkanet root powder – light red to deep purple.

If you don't want to use these natural colors, you can use substitute with ground eye shadow or blush on powder, just put it the final step of the lip balm making method.

Tips of making lip balms.

• If you would prefer a vegan lip balm, you can substitute the beeswax for one of vegan-friendly waxes like Candelillia, Carnauba or Palm wax.

• For a softer balm add an extra tablespoon of a carrier oil of your choice such olive oil, avocado oil, jojoba oil, etc.

• If you don't have the oils listed in these recipes don't worry! You can use another nourishing carrier oils: sweet almond oil, avocado oil, jojoba oil, macadamia nut oil, argan oil, etc.

• One of the benefits of these recipes is that no refrigeration is required. The wax keeps the balm solid in most conditions (avoid heat and to store them in your pants pocket).

• How long should the balm last? It should be fine for approx. 1 year with a natural preservative such as vitamin E. But obvious hygiene precautions should be taken if you're using a pot.

• Always use therapeutic grade for all of the ingredients.

• If you use a recycled container, make sure to clean it thoroughly to prevent bacteria or fungus to contaminate and form in your homemade lip balm.

Cautions about allergies

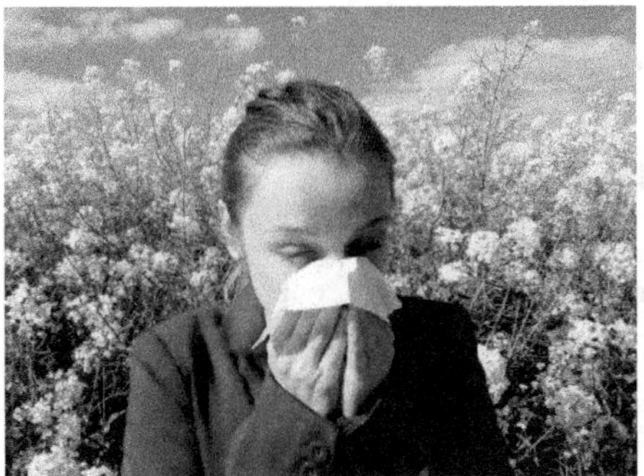

There may be nothing basically wrong with any of the ingredients lip balm manufacturers use for their products, but you personally may have problems with specific ingredients. Suppose you are allergic to paraffin and the ingredient was written in very tiny print on the lip balm packaging? Would you not end up messing your lips more than help them regain their succulence and glossiness? Yet you cannot conclude that you are not going to use lip balms ever.

So, what is the best way out when you do not want to risk off-the-shelf lip balms? It seems a great idea to consider first what, in your case, you wanted lip balm for in the first place. The answer is that with all the dryness and the chapping that coldness occasions on your lips, you wanted to avoid such damage from happening to your lips. You wanted something that would seal the moisture your lips have, right within them. You do not want your lips losing their moisture to the environment, and you do not want any wind that is blowing your way to sweep your lip moisture away.

Storage

You need to think about safe, clean storage. So, sieve the oil and pour it into a clean glass jar in which you are going to store it. Then label the jar appropriately. Next, you need to identify a place that is both cool and dark, and then carefully place your oil jar there. Your oil will be safe as it is for around one year. In case you envisage a situation where your oil is going to last longer than one year, you can choose to store the oil jar in a refrigerator. You just need to remember to let the oil warm up a little before use when you want to make lemon lip balm with it. For this purpose, the oil needs to be at room temperature.

Chapter 2 – **Moisturizing lip balms**

Glossy Peppermint lip balm

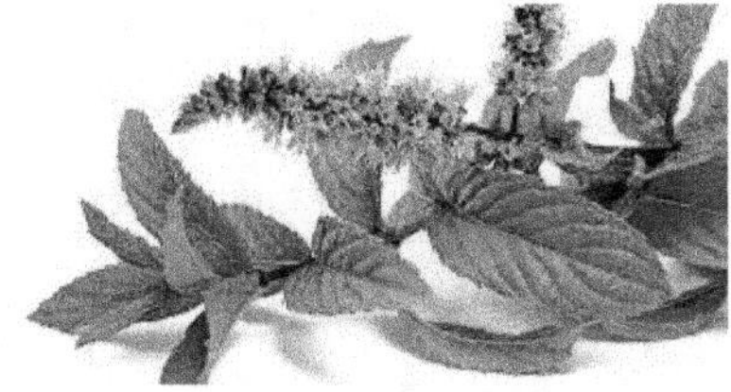

Makes: 3 tins (½ ounce)

Ingredients:

2 teaspoons beeswax pellets

1 teaspoon honey

8 teaspoons jojoba oil

6 drops peppermint essential oil

Preparation steps:

1. If you bought beeswax in block, grate it or chop it with a knife.

2. In a double boiler over medium heat put the beeswax, the honey and the jojoba oil.

3. Stir until it's melted.

4. Remove from heat.

5. Add the peppermint essential oil.

6. Stir again until well combined.

7. Pour the mixture into a lip balm container.

8. Let it cool completely until solid, about 20 minutes.

Glossy Lime lip balm

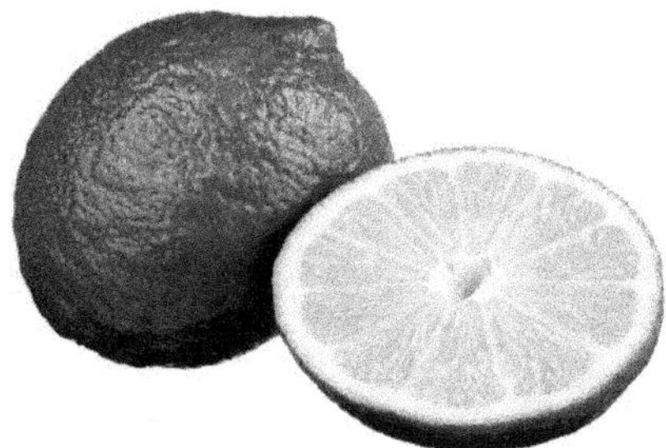

Makes: 3 tins (½ ounce)

Ingredients:

2 teaspoons beeswax pellets

1 teaspoon honey

8 teaspoons jojoba oil

7 drops lime peel essential oil

Preparation steps:

1. If you bought beeswax in block, grate it or chop it with a knife.

2. In a double boiler over medium heat put the beeswax, the honey and the jojoba oil.

3. Stir until it's melted.

4. Remove from heat.

5. Add the lime peel essential oil.

6. Stir again until well combined.

7. Pour the mixture into a lip balm container.

8. Let it cool completely until solid, about 20 minutes.

Glossy Grapefruit lip balm

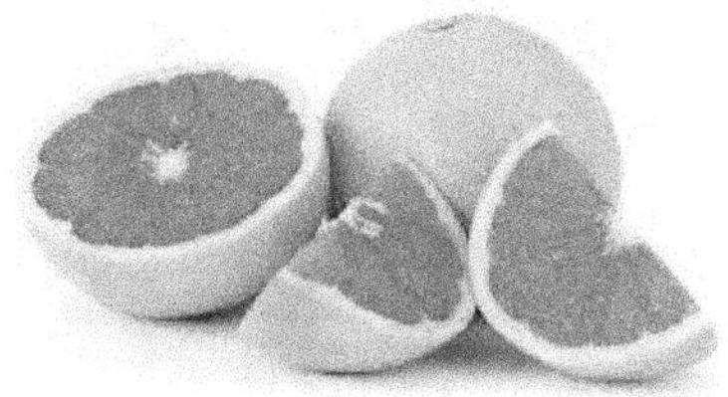

Makes: 3 tins (½ ounce)

Ingredients:

2 teaspoons beeswax pellets

1 teaspoon honey

8 teaspoons sunflower oil

7 drops grapefruit essential oil

Preparation steps:

1. If you bought beeswax in block, grate it or chop it with a knife.

2. In a double boiler over medium heat put the beeswax, the honey and the sunflower oil.

3. Stir until it's melted.

4. Remove from heat.

5. Add the lime grape fruit essential oil.

6. Stir again until well combined.

7. Pour the mixture into a lip balm container.

8. Let it cool completely until solid, about 20 minutes.

Glossy Tangerine lip balm

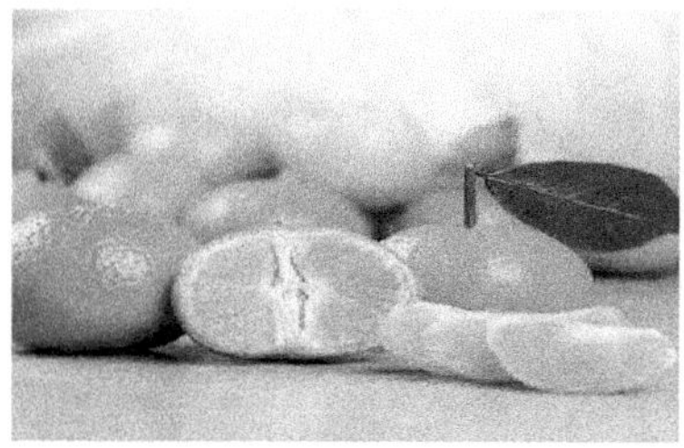

Makes: 3 tins (½ ounce)

Ingredients:

2 teaspoons beeswax pellets

1 teaspoon honey

8 teaspoons jojoba oil

7 drops tangerine essential oil

Preparation steps:

1. If you bought beeswax in block, grate it or chop it with a knife.
2. In a double boiler over medium heat put the beeswax, the honey and the jojoba oil.
3. Stir until it's melted.
4. Remove from heat.
5. Add the lime tangerine essential oil.
6. Stir again until well combined.
7. Pour the mixture into a lip balm container.
8. Let it cool completely until solid, about 20 minutes.

Glossy Lemon lip balm

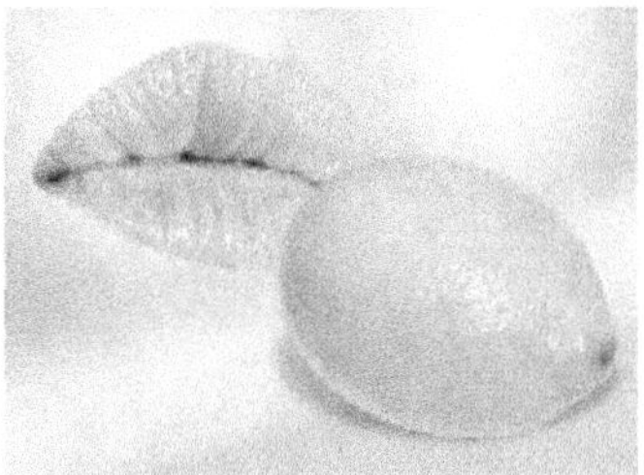

Makes: 3 tins (½ ounce)

Ingredients:

2 teaspoons beeswax pellets
1 teaspoon honey
8 teaspoons sunflower oil
6 drops lemon essential oil

Preparation steps:

1. If you bought beeswax in block, grate it or chop it with a knife.
2. In a double boiler over medium heat put the beeswax, the honey and the sunflower oil.
3. Stir until it's melted.
4. Remove from heat.
5. Add the lime lemon essential oil.
6. Stir again until well combined.
7. Pour the mixture into a lip balm container.
8. Let it cool completely until solid, about 20 minutes.

Chapter 3 – Nourishing lip balms.

Lemon Lip Balm

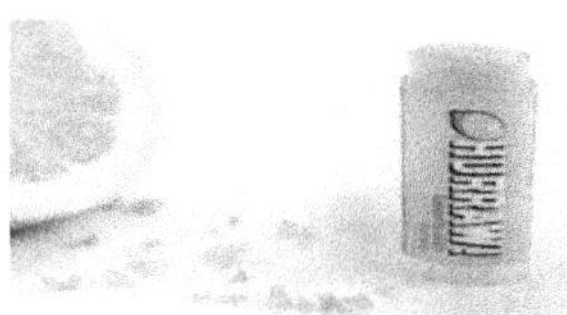

Makes: 3 tins (½ ounce)

Ingredients:

3 teaspoons beeswax pellets

1 teaspoon honey

5 teaspoons sunflower oil

6 drops lemon essential oil

Preparation steps:

1. If you bought beeswax in block, grate it or chop it with a knife.

2. In a double boiler over medium heat put the beeswax, the honey and the sunflower oil.

3. Stir until it's melted.

4. Remove from heat.

5. Add the lime lemon essential oil.

6. Stir again until well combined.

7. Pour the mixture into a lip balm container.

8. Let it cool completely until solid, about 20 minutes.

Lemon chamomile lip balm

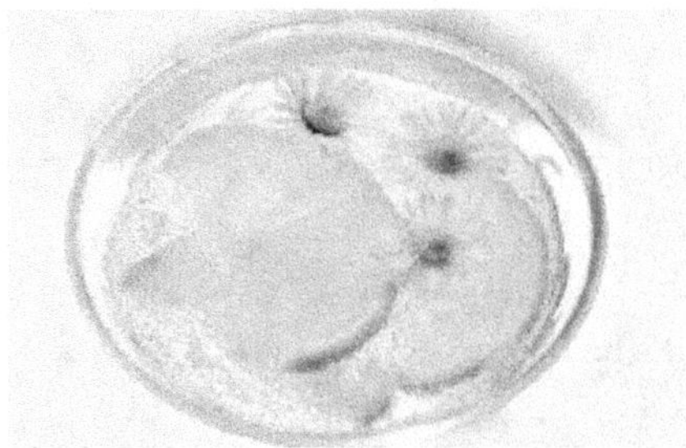

Makes: 15 lip balm tubes 1 ¾ oz.

Ingredients:

2 tablespoons beeswax
2 tablespoons Shea butter
1 tablespoon + 2 teaspoons coconut oil
1 tablespoon chamomile flowers
3 capsules vitamin E
15 drops lemon essential oil

Preparation steps:

1. If you bought beeswax in block, grate it or chop it with a knife.
2. In a double boiler over low-medium heat put ½ cup coconut oil and the chamomile flowers.
3. Cook for at least 1 hour.
4. Then strain through a coffee filter, but beware, it's very hot!
5. Put the mixture into a jar and take 1 tablespoon + 2 teaspoons of it.

6. Put it into a double boiler over a medium heat with the beeswax and the Shea butter.

7. Stir until it's melted.

8. Remove from heat.

9. Add the vitamin E oil and the lemon essential oil.

10. Stir again until well combined.

11. Pour the mixture into a lip balm tubes.

12. Let it cool completely until solid, about 2 hours.

Lemon Rosemary Shinny Lip Balm

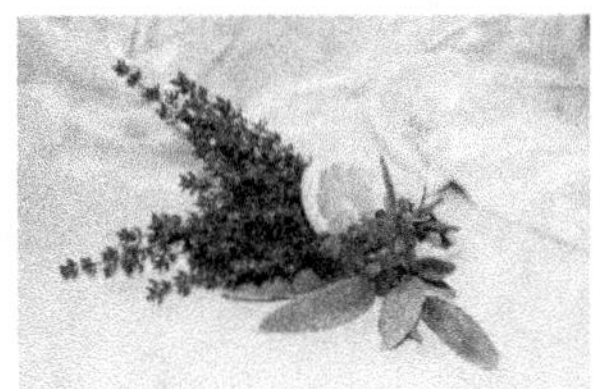

Makes: 12 tins

Ingredients:

2 tablespoons beeswax pellets

½ cup almond oil (or olive oil)

A slice of pink colored organic lip stick

15 drops lemon essential oil

15 drops rosemary essential oil

3 capsules vitamin E oil

Preparation steps:

1. If you bought beeswax in block, grate it or chop it with a knife.

2. In a double boiler over medium heat put the beeswax, the almond oil and the slice of lip stick.

3. Stir until it's melted.

4. Remove from heat.

5. Add the vitamin E oil, the lemon essential oil and the rosemary essential oil.

6. Stir again until well combined.

7. Pour the mixture into a lip balm tubes.

8. Let it cool completely until solid, about 2 hours.

Peppermint Lip Balm

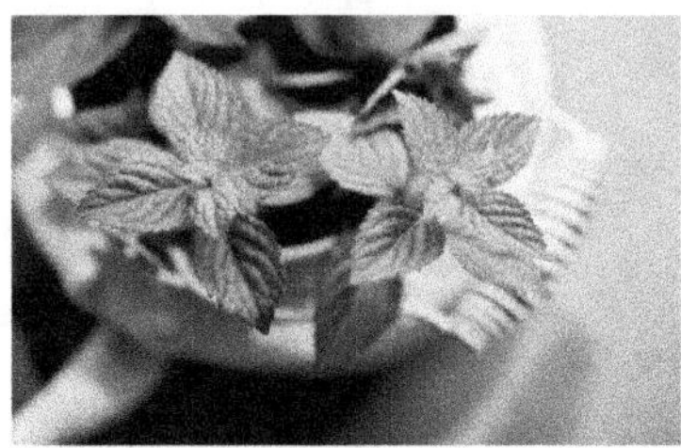

Makes: 3 tins (½ ounce)

Ingredients:

3 teaspoons beeswax pellets
1 teaspoon honey
5 teaspoons jojoba oil
6 drops peppermint essential oil

Preparation steps:

1. If you bought beeswax in block, grate it or chop it with a knife.
2. In a double boiler over medium heat put the beeswax, the honey and the jojoba oil.
3. Stir until it's melted.
4. Remove from heat.
5. Add the peppermint essential oil.
6. Stir again until well combined.
7. Pour the mixture into a lip balm container.
8. Let it cool completely until solid, about 20 minutes.

Peppermint - Mocha Lip Gloss

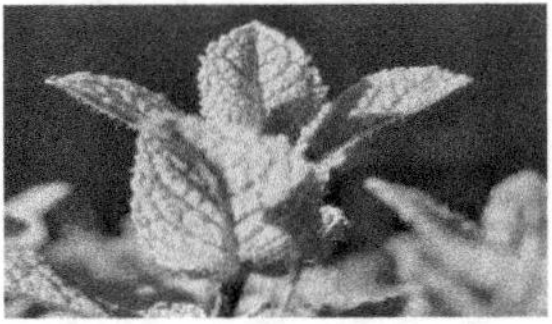

Makes: 10-12 tins

Ingredients:

· 0,5 oz. beeswax pellets
· 0,5 oz. Shea butter
· 0,5 oz. avocado oil (or olive oil)
· 0,4 oz. sweet almond oil
· 0,2 oz. castor oil
· 1 teaspoon cocoa powder
· 8 drops peppermint essential oïl
· 1 capsule vitamin E oil

Preparation steps:

1. If you bought beeswax in block, grate it or chop it with a knife.
2. In a double boiler over medium heat put the beeswax, the Shea butter and the oils.
3. Stir until it's melted.
4. Remove from heat.
5. Add the cocoa powder, the peppermint essential oil and the vitamin E oil.
6. Stir again until well combined.
7. Pour the mixture into a lip balm tubes.
8. Let it cool completely until solid, about 2 hours.

Tangerine Lip Balm

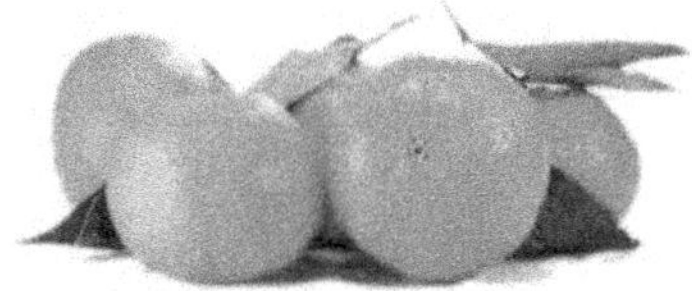

Makes: 3 tins (½ ounce)

Ingredients:

3 teaspoons beeswax pellets
1 teaspoon honey
5 teaspoons jojoba oil
7 drops tangerine essential oil

Preparation steps:

1. If you bought beeswax in block, grate it or chop it with a knife.
2. In a double boiler over medium heat put the beeswax, the honey and the jojoba oil.
3. Stir until it's melted.
4. Remove from heat.
5. Add the lime tangerine essential oil.
6. Stir again until well combined.
7. Pour the mixture into a lip balm container.
8. Let it cool completely until solid, about 20 minutes.

Coconut Rose Lip Balm

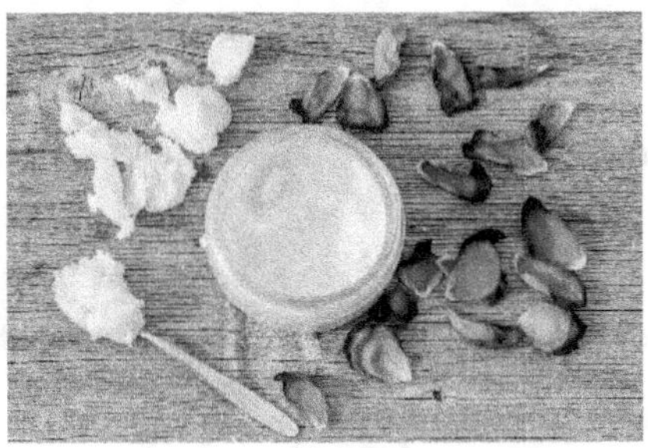

Makes: 6 lip balm containers

Ingredients:

1/4 cup Beeswax

1/4 cup Rose Petals (fresh or dried)

1/8 cup Shea Butter

1/8 cup Coconut Oil

1 teaspoon Coconut essential oil

1 teaspoon Sweet Almond Oil

Preparation steps:

1. If you bought beeswax in block, grate it or chop it with a knife.

2. In a double boiler over medium heat put the beeswax, the Shea butter, and the coconut oil.

3. Stir until it's melted.

4. Add the Rose petals.

5. Stir until well combined.

6. Remove from heat.

7. Add the coconut essential oil and the almond oil.

8. Stir again until well combined.

9. Strain the rose petals.

10. Pour the mixture into a lip balm container.

11. Let it cool completely until solid, about 2 hours.

Quick tip: You can leave rose petals in the mixture or strain them, it's up to you.

Grapefruit Lip Balm

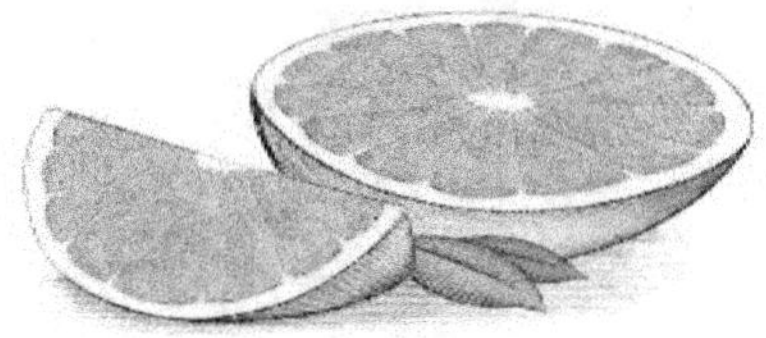

Makes: 3 tins (½ ounce)

Ingredients:

3 teaspoons beeswax pellets

1 teaspoon honey

5 teaspoons sunflower oil

7 drops grapefruit essential oil

Preparation steps:

1. If you bought beeswax in block, grate it or chop it with a knife.

2. In a double boiler over medium heat put the beeswax, the honey and the sunflower oil.

3. Stir until it's melted.

4. Remove from heat.

5. Add the lime grape fruit essential oil.

6. Stir again until well combined.

7. Pour the mixture into a lip balm container.

8. Let it cool completely until solid, about 20 minutes.

Coconut – Vanilla - Rose Lip Balm

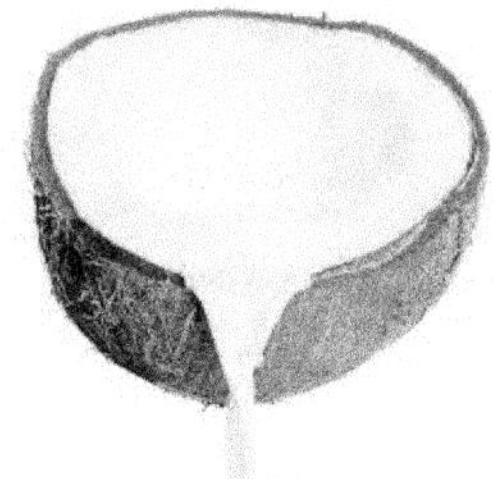

Makes: 6 lip balm containers

Ingredients:

1/4 cup Beeswax

1/4 cup Rose Petals (fresh or dried)

1/8 cup Shea Butter

1/8 cup Coconut Oil

1 teaspoon Vanilla essential oil

1 teaspoon Sweet Almond Oil

Preparation steps:

1. If you bought beeswax in block, grate it or chop it with a knife.

2. In a double boiler over medium heat put the beeswax, the Shea butter, and the coconut oil.

3. Stir until it's melted.

4. Add the Rose petals.

5. Stir until well combined.

6. Remove from heat.

7. Add the vanilla essential oil and the almond oil.

8. Stir again until well combined.

9. Strain the rose petals.

10. Pour the mixture into a lip balm container.

11. Let it cool completely until solid, about 2 hours.

Quick tip: You can leave rose petals in the mixture or strain them, it's up to you.

Coconut & Tea Tree Oil Lip Balm

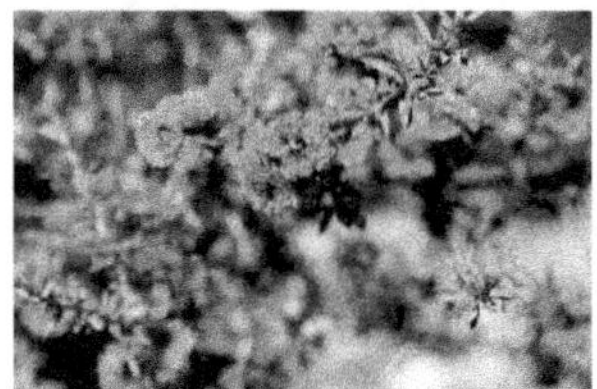

Makes: Approx. 20 tins

Ingredients:

· 1 cup beeswax pellets

· 3 tablespoon coconut oil

· 1 teaspoon vitamin E oil (or 4 capsules)

· 3 drops tea tree oil

Preparation steps:

1. If you bought beeswax in block, grate it or chop it with a knife.
2. In a double boiler over medium heat put the beeswax and the coconut oil.
3. Stir until it's melted.
4. Remove from heat.
5. Add the vitamin E and the tea tree oil.
6. Stir again until well combined.
7. Pour the mixture into a lip balm container.
8. Let it cool completely until solid, about 2 hours.

Quick tip: Yes it's a huge quantity of lip balm, but it's a wonderful gift!

Vanilla - Cocoa Smooth Lip Balm Recipe

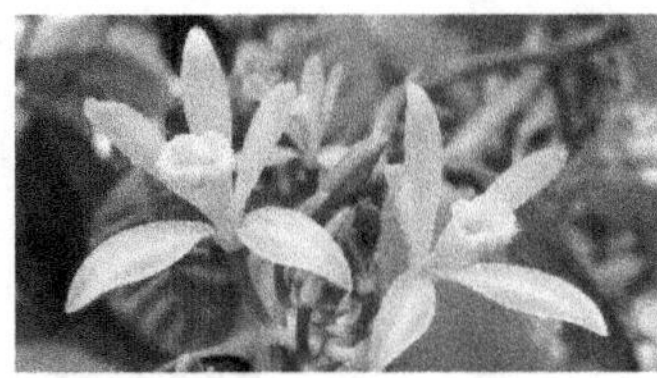

Makes: 12 tins

Ingredients:

· 1 ½ oz. beeswax pellets

· 1 oz. almond oil

· 1 oz. aloe oil

· 1/2 oz. cocoa butter

· 1/2 oz. Shea butter

· 1/2 oz. jojoba oil

· 1/2 oz. avocado oil

· 4 capsules vitamin E oil

· ¾ teaspoon vanilla extract

Preparation steps:

1. If you bought beeswax in block, grate it or chop it with a knife.
2. In a double boiler over medium heat put the beeswax, the butters and the oils.
3. Stir until it's melted.
4. Remove from heat.
5. Add the vitamin E oil and the vanilla extract.
6. Stir again until well combined.
7. Pour the mixture into lip balm containers.

Vanilla-White Chocolate lip balm

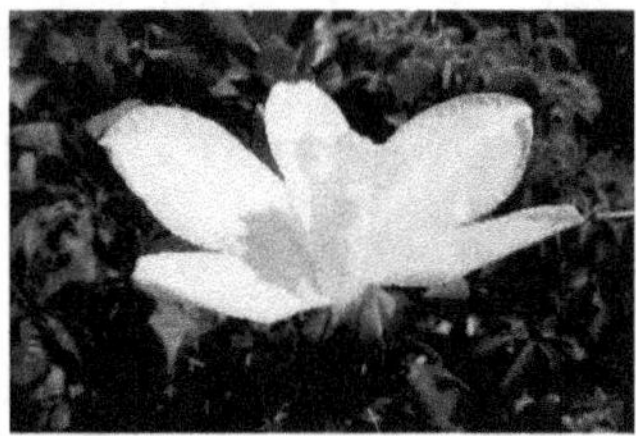

Makes: 4 tins

Ingredients:

· 1 tsp. Honey · 1 tsp. Olive oil
· 1 tsp. Almond oil
· 1 tbsp. Shea butter
· 1 tbsp. Beeswax pellets
· 5 white Chocolate chips
· 4 drops Vanilla essential oil

Preparation steps

1. In a double boiler over medium heat put the honey, the oils, the beeswax, the chocolate chips and the Shea butter.
2. Stir until it's melted.
3. Remove from heat and add the Vanilla essential oil.
4. Stir again.
5. Pour the mixture into lip gloss containers.
6. Let them cool completely until solid, about 20 minutes.

Quick tip:Use only white chocolate, using other chocolate types are not a good idea.

Vanilla-White Chocolate lip balm

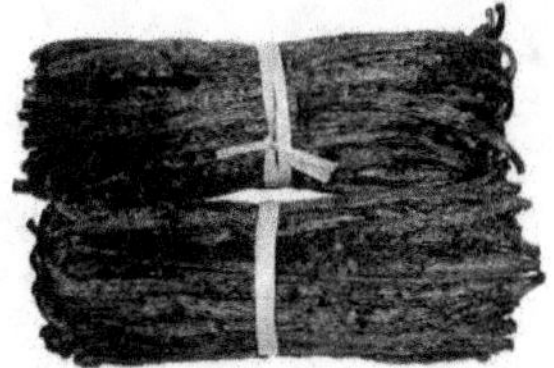

Makes: 4 tins

Ingredients:

· 1 tsp. Honey · 1 tsp. Olive oil
· 1 tsp. Almond oil
· 1 tbsp. Shea butter
· 1 tbsp. Beeswax pellets
· 5 white Chocolate chips
· 4 drops Vanilla essential oil
· A pinch Oatmeal
· A pinch dry whole milk

Preparation steps

1. In a double boiler over medium heat put the honey, the oils, the beeswax, the chocolate chips and the Shea butter.
2. Stir until it's melted.
3. Remove from heat and add the Vanilla essential oil.
4. Stir again.
5. Add in the dry milk and the oatmeal.
6. Stir until well combined.
7. Pour the mixture into lip gloss containers.
8. Let them cool completely until solid, about 20 minutes.

Vanilla Latte Lip Balm

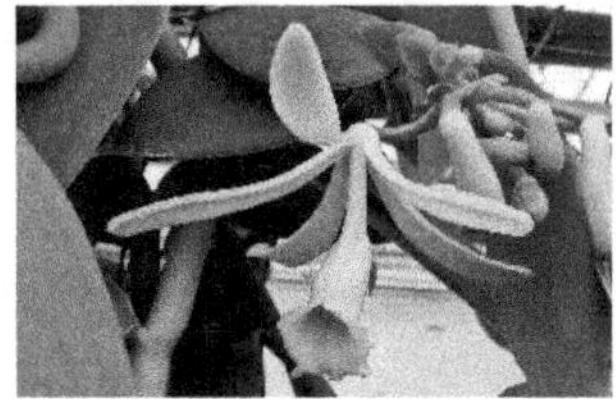

Makes: 20 lip balm containers

Ingredients:

· 4 oz. Cocoa Butter
· 2 oz. Coffee infused almond oil (see above)
· .6 oz. Avocado Oil
· 1 tablespoon vanilla extract
· A pinch of sugar

Preparation steps:

1. If you bought beeswax in block, grate it or chop it with a knife.
2. In a double boiler over medium heat put the cocoa butter, the avocado oil and the coffee infused oil.
3. Stir until it's melted.
4. Add the sugar and stir until it's fully dissolved.
5. Remove from heat.
6. Add the vanilla extract.
7. Stir again until well combined.
8. Pour the mixture into a lip balm tubes.
9. Let it cool completely until solid, about 2 hours.

Quick tip: The Vanilla extract is optional. Without it the lip balm tastes like a cup of black coffee.

Vanilla Lip Balm

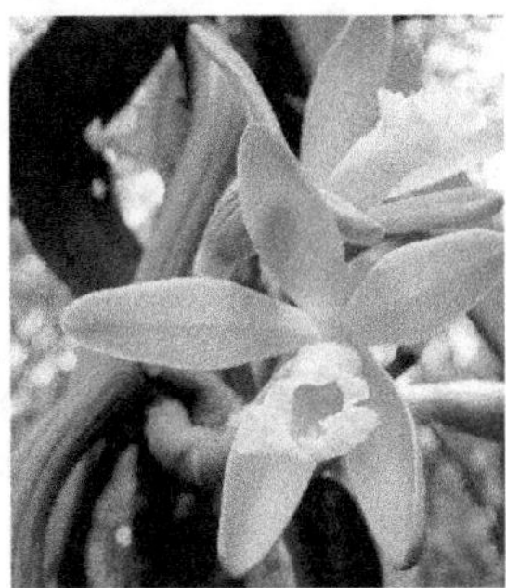

Makes: 3 containers

Ingredients:

· 1 tablespoon coconut oil
· 1 tablespoon beeswax pellets
· 1 capsule vitamin E oil
· 1/8 teaspoon vanilla extract

Preparation steps:

1. If you bought beeswax in block, grate it or chop it with a knife.
2. In a double boiler over medium heat put the coconut oil and the beeswax.
3. Stir until it's melted.
4. Remove from heat.
5. Add the vitamin E and the vanilla extract.
6. Stir again until well combined.
7. Pour the mixture into lip balm tubes.
Let it cool completely until solid, about 1 hour.

Chapter 4 – Regenerating lip balms

Chocolate Covered Orange Lip Balm

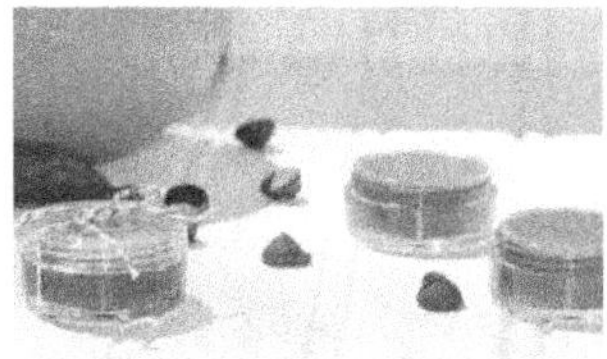

Makes: 6 tins

Ingredients:

- · 2 Tablespoons Almond Oil (or Olive Oil)
- · 1 Tablespoon + 1 teaspoon beeswax pellets
- · 1 Tablespoon Cocoa Butter
- · 1 Tablespoon Coconut Oil
- · 10 semi-sweet chocolate chips
- · 8 drops Sweet Orange Essential Oil
- · 1 capsule Vitamin E oil

Preparation steps:

1. If you bought beeswax in block, grate it or chop it with a knife.
2. In a double boiler over medium heat put the beeswax, the almond oil, the cocoa butter and the coconut oil.
3. Stir until it's melted.
4. Remove from heat.
5. Add the chocolate chips, the sweet orange essential oils and the vitamin E oil.
6. Stir again until well combined.
7. Pour the mixture into a lip balm tubes.
8. Let it cool completely until solid, about 2 hours.

Homemade Coffee Flavored Lip Balm Recipe

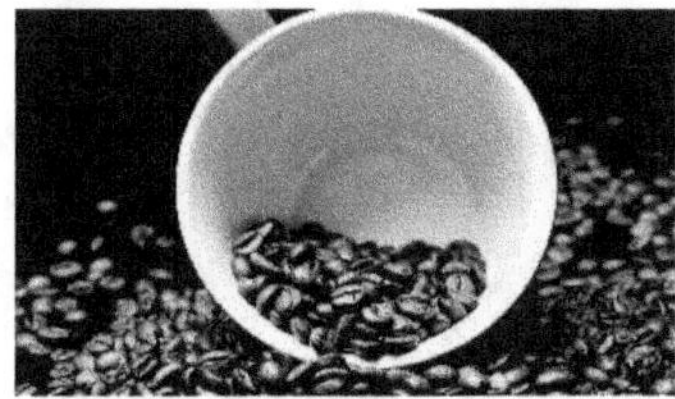

Makes: 10 tins

Ingredients:

· 1 oz. olive oil (see above)
· .5 oz. cocoa butter
· .5 oz. Shea butter
· .25 oz. beeswax pellets
· 1/2 ml Chocolate Devil's Food Cake flavor oil
· 1/2 ml Kahlua flavor oil
· 10 drops clove essential oil
· A pinch of sugar

Preparation steps:

1. If you bought beeswax in block, grate it or chop it with a knife.
2. In a double boiler over medium heat put the beeswax, the olive oil, the cocoa butter and the Shea butter.
3. Stir until it's melted.
4. Add a pinch of sugar and stir until fully dissolved.
5. Remove from heat.
6. Add the clove essential oil and the flavors.
7. Stir again until well combined.
8. Pour the mixture into a lip balm tubes.
9. Let it cool completely until solid, about 2 hours.

DIY Mocha Lip Balm

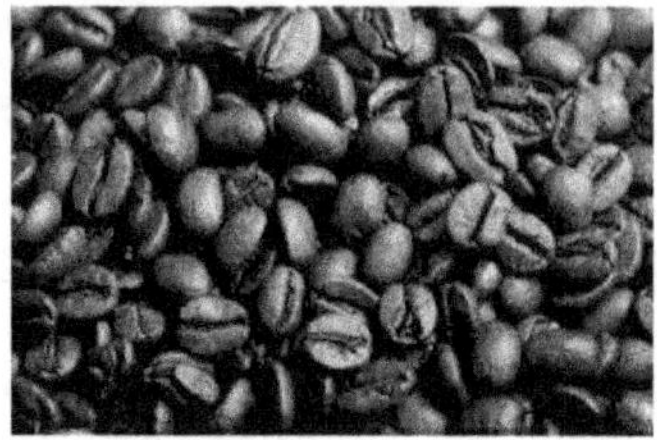

Makes: 9 lip balm tubes

Ingredients:

· 0,7 oz. coffee-infused almond oil

· 0,4 oz. coconut oil

· 0,35 oz. cocoa butter

· 0,3 oz. beeswax pellets

· 2 drops cocoa flavor

Preparation steps:

1. If you bought beeswax in block, grate it or chop it with a knife.
2. In a double boiler over medium heat put the beeswax, the coconut oil, the cocoa butter and the coffee infused oil.
3. Stir until it's melted.
4. Remove from heat.
5. Add the flavor.
6. Stir again until well combined.
7. Pour the mixture into a lip balm tubes.
8. Let it cool completely until solid, about 2 hours.

Clove and orange lip balm

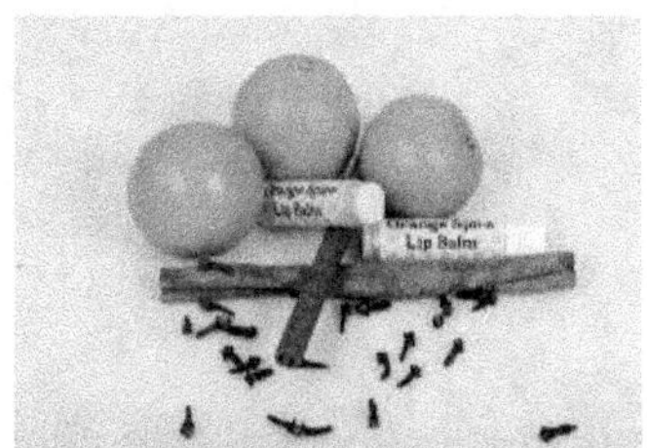

Makes: 12 tubes

Ingredients:

1 tablespoon + 1 teaspoon Beeswax pellets

3 tablespoons Sunflower Oil (or *Almond* oil)

1 tablespoon Shea Butter

25 drops Sweet Orange essential oil

5 drops Clove essential oil

Preparation steps:

1. If you bought beeswax in block, grate it or chop it with a knife.

2. In a double boiler over medium heat put the beeswax, the sunflower oil and the Shea butter.

3. Stir until it's melted.

4. Remove from heat.

5. Add the sweet orange and clove essential oils.

6. Stir again until well combined.

7. Pour the mixture into a lip balm tubes.

8. Let it cool completely until solid, about 20 minutes.

Coffee almond oil infused

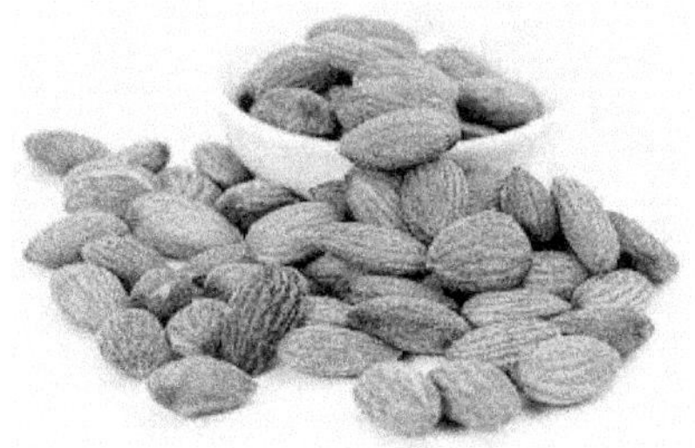

Ingredients

· 3 tablespoon coffee ground
· 4 oz. almond oil

Preparation

1. Blend coffee beans for a few seconds then place them in a coffee filter.
2. Close the coffee filter with a string.
3. Put it in a jar.
4. Cover with the almond oil.
5. Close the jar.
6. Let it infuse for 2 weeks.

Almond Shea lip butter

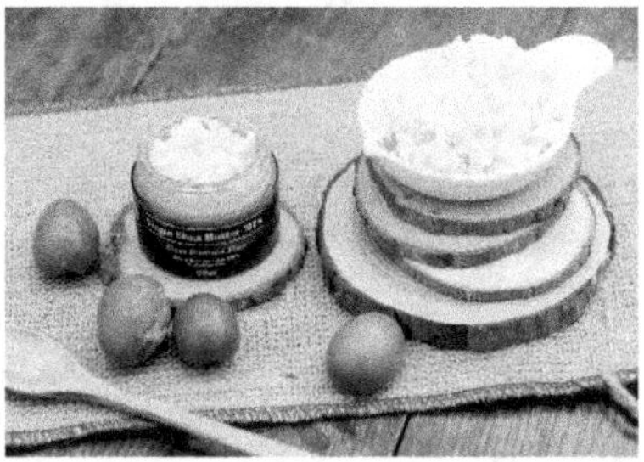

Makes: 5 tins

Ingredients:

1,4 oz. Shea butter
0,35 oz. sweet almond oil

Preparation steps:

1. In a double boiler over medium heat put the Shea butter and the almond oil.
2. Stir until it's melted.
3. Remove from heat.
4. Pour the mixture into a lip balm tubes.
5. Let it cool completely until solid, about 20 minutes.

Good Night Kiss Lip Balm

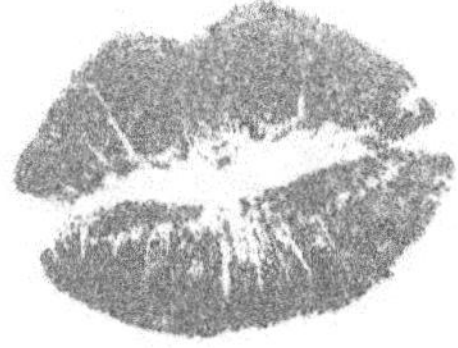

Makes: 6 lip balm pots - 1,5 oz.

Ingredients:

2 tablespoons beeswax pellets
1 tablespoon Mango butter
1 tablespoon Shae butter
1 tablespoon Sweet Almond Oil
½ tablespoon cocoa butter
½ tablespoon honey
12 drops peppermint essential oil
8 drops vanilla essential oil
6 drops cinnamon bark essential oil

Preparation steps:

1. If you bought beeswax in block, grate it or chop it with a knife.
2. In a double boiler over medium heat put the beeswax, the Shea butter, the cocoa butter and the mango butter.
3. Stir until it's melted.
4. Add the honey and the almond oil.

5. Stir until it's well combined.

6. Remove from heat.

7. Add the essential oils.

8. Stir again until well combined.

9. Pour the mixture into a lip balm pots.

10. Let it cool completely until solid, about 2 hours.

Quick tip: When pouring the lip balm pots, if the mixture hardens, put it back on the double boiler for a few seconds

Rose Geranium Lip Balm

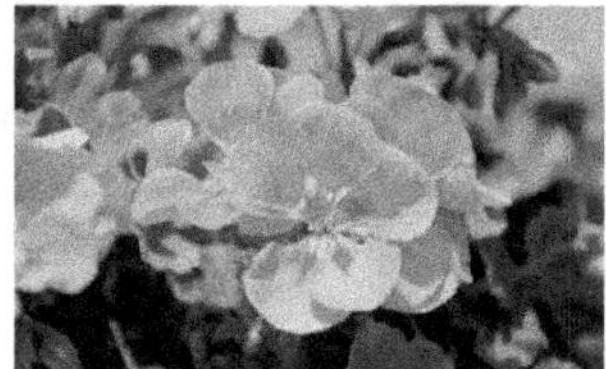

Makes: 4 tins

Ingredients:

0,5 oz. avocado oil

0,5 oz. Shea butter

0,4 oz. beeswax pellets

2 capsules Vitamin E oil

5 drops rose geranium essential oil

Preparation steps:

1. If you bought beeswax in block, grate it or chop it with a knife.
2. In a double boiler over medium heat put the beeswax and the avocado oil.
3. Stir until it's melted.
4. Remove from heat.
5. Add the rose geranium essential oil and the vitamin E.
6. Stir again until well combined.
7. Pour the mixture into a lip balm pots.
8. Let it cool completely until solid, about 2 hours.

Quick tip: When pouring the lip balm pots, if the mixture hardens, put it back on the double boiler for a few seconds.

Bronze Goddess Tinted Lip balm Recipe

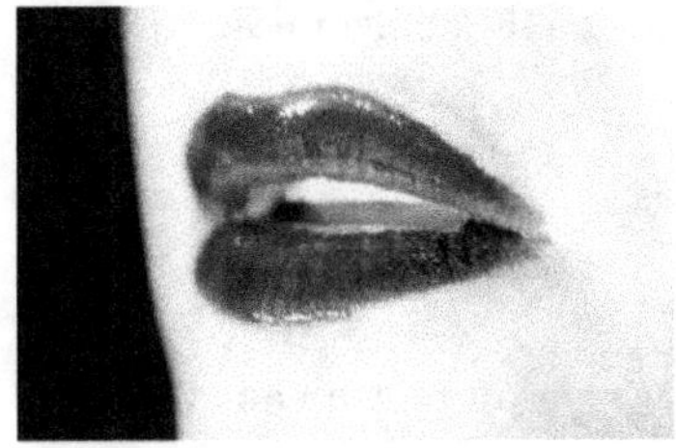

Makes: 4 tins

Ingredients:

· 2 1/2 teaspoons coconut oil
· 2 teaspoons beeswax
· 1 1/2 teaspoons sweet almond oil
· 1 teaspoon mango butter
· 1 teaspoon kukui nut oil
· 1 teaspoon aloe vera oil
· 1/2 teaspoon cocoa butter
· 1/2 teaspoon vitamin E oil
· 1/4 teaspoon amber mica
· 12 drops Brown sugar Flavor oil

Preparation steps:

1. If you bought beeswax in block, grate it or chop it with a knife.
2. In a double boiler over medium heat put the coconut oil, the beeswax, the almond oil, the mango butter, the kukui oil, the aloe vera oil and the cocoa butter.

3. Stir until it's melted.

4. Remove from heat.

5. Add the brown sugar flavor oil, the vitamin E oil and the amber mica.

6. Stir again until well combined.

7. Pour the mixture into lip balm containers.

8. Let it cool completely until solid, about 2 hours.

Quick tip: Basically you can substitute brown sugar flavor oil with any flavor oil you want, make your own experiences!

Hemp & Honey Lip Balm

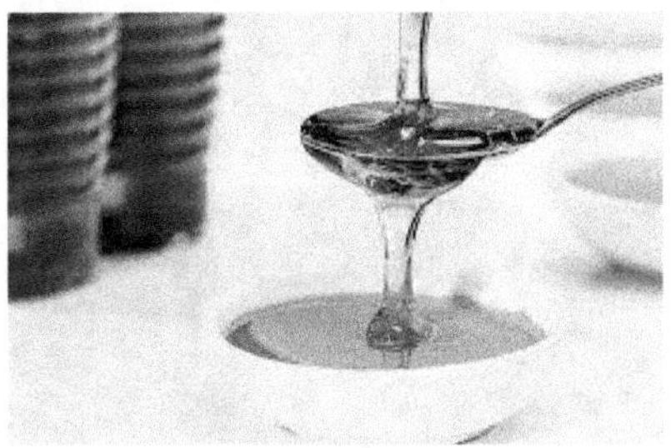

Makes: 12 lip balm tubes or 4 lip balm containers

Ingredients:

· ½ oz. beeswax pellets
· 1/3 oz. cocoa butter
· 1/3 oz. carnauba wax
· 0,18 oz. Shea butter
· 1 tablespoon + 1 teaspoon almond oil
· 2 teaspoons honey
· 1 teaspoon hemp oil
· 8 drops citrus essential oil

Preparation steps:

1. If you bought beeswax in block, grate it or chop it with a knife.
2. In a double boiler over medium heat put the beeswax, the cocoa butter, the carnauba wax and the almond oil.
3. Stir until it's melted.

4. Add the hemp oil and the honey.

5. Mix with a milk frother (because the honey doesn't mix well in the oil) until well combined

6. Remove from heat.

7. Add the citrus essential oil.

8. Stir again until well combined.

9. Pour the mixture into a lip balm container.

10. Let it cool completely until solid, about 2 hours.

Quick tip: The recipes could look like pretty complicated with all the ingredients to weight out, but trust me, you won't r

Conclusion.

Lip balm is used when someone has angular cheilitis or stomatitis; or is just suffering from cold sores. Incidentally, what is this cheilitis? Well, it is another term given to chapping of lips, only this time the chapping is significantly severe. In fact, you get to see real cracks around your lip corners. Sometimes, however, cheilitis is caused by infection, and so if your lip balm does not seem to work, you better ask your doctor what the heck is happening to your lips. In short, we are saying here that lip balm, lovely as it is for your comfort and beauty, is not a substitute for medication.

Bonus Chapter

Advantages of Lip Scrub

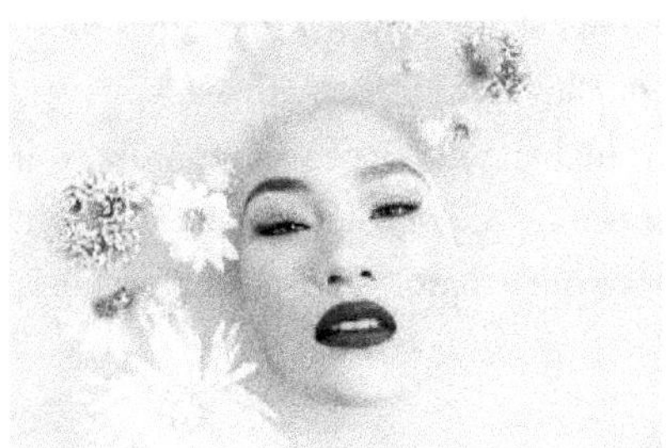

When you remove the dead skin from your lips (and yes, it IS skin – just a different type than on the rest of your body), it helps in bringing out the fresh, new layers. This will make your lips smooth, soft, and, of course – kissable! That's a great benefit, but it's not the only one.

When your lips have a smooth surface, your cosmetics will adhere to them longer. This makes your DIY lip balm and lip gloss more long lasting and effective.

Exfoliating your lips makes them moister, and helps them to retain that moisture. This prevents cracked lips.

If you regularly use lip scrubs, you won't have to worry about the cold or wind causing you to get chapped lips. Apply a DIY lip scrub and you'll be moisturized and good to go.

Using a Lip Scrub

Beauty and health experts recommend using a lip scrub once a week or more. You may need to do it more frequently during the dry winter months. It just takes several minutes to do a lip scrub, so it's easy to add to your routine once a week, or as needed.

Beauty and cosmetic shops carry lip scrub products. But if you want a healthier, less expensive option, then you can make them easily at home. In fact, you probably have most of the ingredients in your pantry already.

You should only put products on your lips that are known to be safe, and that will not be likely to cause allergic reactions. If you accidentally ingest some of your DIY scrub, it's not usually a problem at all.

Sugar Coconut DIY Lip Scrub

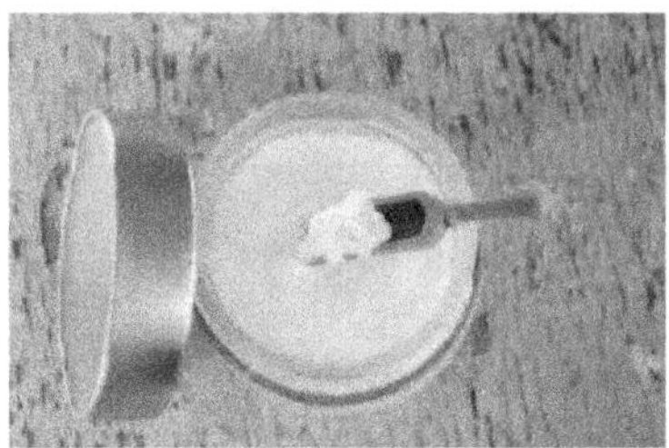

Ingredients

1 tablespoon of organic honey

2 tablespoons of coconut sugar

2 tablespoons of melted coconut oil

Preparation steps:

Combine all the helpful ingredients above in a small bowl until they are fully combined. This creates a grainy, thick scrub, which is exactly what you want for exfoliation. It stores well in your refrigerator for up to three weeks.

Usage

Use about 1/4 teaspoon of the coconut sugar DIY lip scrub and apply to dry lips. Massage the scrub in a circular motion, on your lips and around the lip area. Don't use harsh pressure, but rather gentle circles. This will still give you exfoliation benefits.

Rinse your lips with water and pat them dry. Follow it with your favorite lip balm or moisturizer.

Ginger Snap Edible Lip Scrub

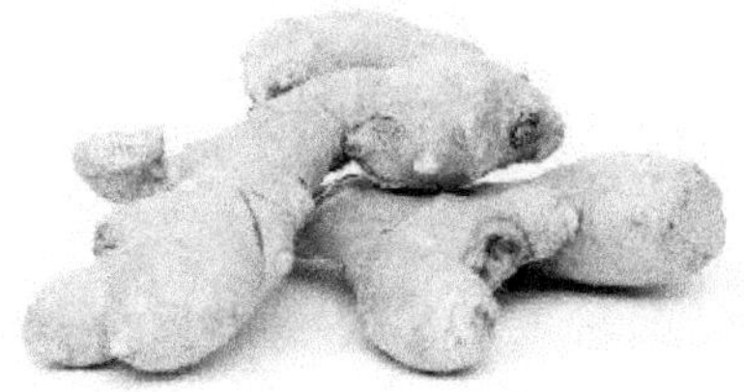

Ingredients

A pinch of cinnamon, ground 1/2 teaspoon of ginger, ground 1 teaspoon of coconut oil, melted, virgin

1 teaspoon of organic maple syrup

1/4 cup of corn meal

1/4 cup of brown sugar, vegan

Preparation steps:

Combine the ingredients above until they are well-mixed. Place the mixture in one medium container or a set of smaller ones.

Usage

Using the Ginger Snap Edible Lip Scrub is easy and quick. Moisten your lips and massage a dime-sized amount of lip scrub in circular, small motions for one to two minutes. Allow the mixture to remain on your lips for a minute or so. Then rinse with warm water (or lick!) to remove the scrub. Pat the lips dry and then apply your favorite DIY lip balm.

Avocado Oil DIY Lip Scrub

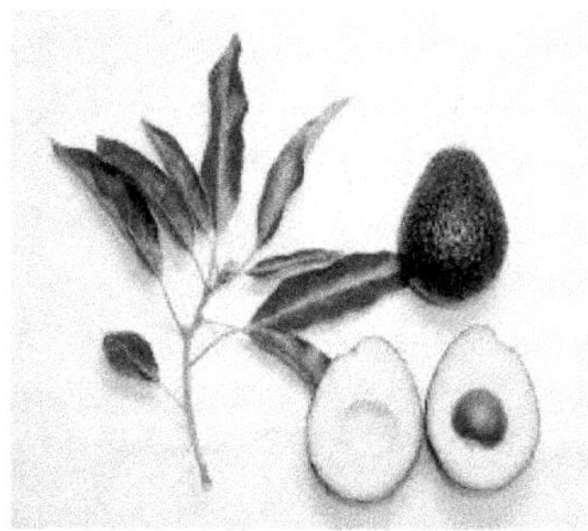

Ingredients

1/2 ounce of avocado oil

3/4 ounce of yellow beeswax

1/4 ounce of vitamin E oil

3/4 ounce of almond oil, sweet

2 & 1/2 ounces of white sugar

1 ounce of Shea butter

1/4 ounce of buttercream flavoring

Preparation steps:

1.   Combine the liquid oils, beeswax and Shea butter in a Pyrex-type glass measuring cup. Heat in the microwave until beeswax melts completely, 30 seconds at a time.

2.   Once all oils are liquefied, stir in your favorite flavored oil & natural sweetener. Whisk to mix fully.

3.   Stir in the 2 & 1/2 ounces of sugar. Pour in containers and allow to harden.

Usage

Using your finger, apply about 1/4 of a teaspoon full of scrub on your lips. Rub in circular motions for about 30 seconds. You can go a bit longer if you need exfoliation particularly badly. Wipe off scrub with a damp washcloth and then apply DIY lip balm. This will leave your lips feeling silky and smooth!

Cinnamon Honey Lip Scrub

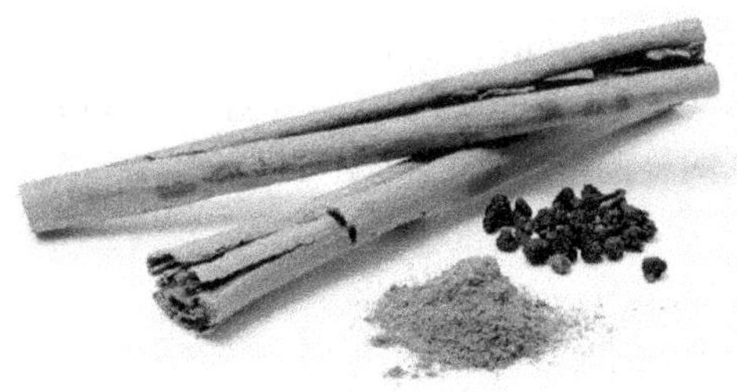

Ingredients

2 ounces of brown sugar (regular sugar is OK, but brown sugar tastes better)
1 teaspoon of cinnamon powder (or cloves, ginger powder or nutmeg) 1 tablespoon of honey, raw, unfiltered
1 tablespoon of coconut, olive or almond oil

Preparation steps:

1.   Combine your ingredients together in a bowl. Transfer to a lidded jar.
2.   Rub just a small amount of scrub on your lips using circular motions for one to two minutes. Lick the mixture off or wipe with a warm washcloth. Use a DIY lip balm to help lock in the moisture.

Edible Fruit & Sugar Lip Scrub

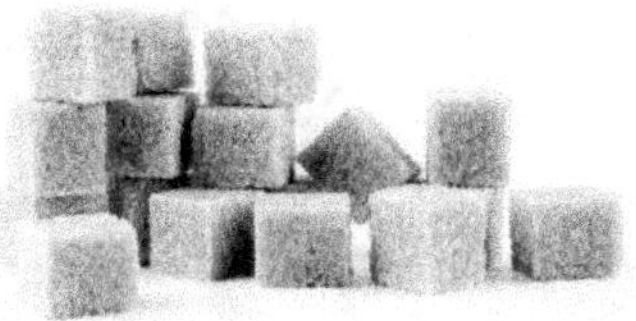

Ingredients

1 teaspoon of honey

1 teaspoon of brown sugar

1 teaspoon of coconut or olive oil

Optional: 1 teaspoon of almond extract

Preparation steps:

1. Mix the ingredients until the consistency is like paste.

2. For exfoliation, apply and rub on lips for at least a half a minute. Lick to remove. Be sure to moisturize your lips after you exfoliate them.

3. Continue to scrub once a week or once every few days if your lips are very dry and chapped. Always moisturize after exfoliating.

9 781979 875912